The Ayahuasca Guidebook

The Sacred *Dieta* & Ceremony Preparation Tips
For the Best Experience Possible

The Ayahuasca Guidebook

The Sacred *Dieta* & Ceremony Preparation Tips
For the Best Experience Possible

Sharon C. Davis

SACRED MEDICINE
—— PRESS ——

2019

The Ayahuasca Guidebook: The Sacred *Dieta* & Ceremony Preparation Tips for the Best Experience Possible. © 2019 by Sharon C. Davis. All rights reserved.

First Edition
First Printing, 2019

Cover design by Sharon C. Davis
www.exposedpixel.com

ISBN 978-0-359-27813-8

Sacred Medicine Press
14500 E. 14th Street #3345
San Leandro, California 94578

www.sacredmedicinepress.com

Ordering Information:
Special discounts are available on quantity purchases by associations, educators, and others. For details, contact the publisher at the above listed address.

U.S. Trade bookstores and wholesalers
Please contact:
Sacred Medicine Press
Tel: (925) 708-9520
Email: exposedpixel@gmail.com

Dedication

This book is dedicated to the sacred and powerful healing plant native to Peru, *La Madre* Ayahausca. All the words in this book stem from the ancient healing space I have shared with her.

I prayed for her guidance with each word on these pages to bring each of you the greatest wisdom of working with this powerful medicine so you may stay safe and be able to access the profound healing and highest teachings possible.

When Ayahuasca is used in the right way, the deepest regions of your mind and soul become cleansed with love, truth, and awareness; allowing you to open your heart and access the ability to heal yourself.

We are all one. The healing you receive ultimately reaches out to all those around you and to the soul of *La Madre* Earth, who needs us now more than ever.

May the truth set you *free.*

Contents

Foreword

So, you feel the call to work with Madre Ayahuasca. The jungle beckons with all its secrets and so too does the Sacred Valley of Peru where the living mysteries want to be known.

But where should you go? With whom should you sit? What should you look for with a *curandero* (shaman) and a lodge? What IS it about plant medicine anyway and what is the best way to prepare for it?

The *Ayahuasca Guidebook* asks the questions you should ask and knows the answers you will find. It covers a weekly countdown for the *sacred dieta protocol, the spiritual dieta, how to overcome fear, supportive plants, integration, a packing guide, travel tips* and so much more.

Sharon Davis' handy book is an invaluable guide to navigating the practicalities of the Peruvian Ayahuasca scene, so you can find that sacred healing space you are seeking within.

Rak Razam
Author/Producer
www.aya-awakenings.com

Seek and You Shall Find

Prior to my first Ayahuasca Ceremony, I was given a brief list of the Sacred *Dieta,* which consisted of a list of foods and medications to avoid before drinking the Ayahuasca brew. After extensive research, I found there was much more preparation than I had anticipated. I also found inconsistencies in the Sacred *Dieta* from one retreat to the next; some leaving out important details, which I later found to be life-threatening when mixed with Ayahuasca.

Many people in our Ayahuasca circle expressed the desire for a more detailed, accurate, and easy to follow information guide regarding the very strict dietary requirements of the Sacred *Dieta*, as well as how to prepare spiritually in the weeks leading up to ceremony.

It is stressful enough, especially as a newcomer, to dive into a life-changing experience without the added worry about which foods and/or medications to cut out prior to doing this plant medicine safely. Feeling safe is the number one priority when doing this medicine; concerns were also brought forth about if they were in the right place or with the right shaman.

Most people who participate in Ayahuasca ceremonies do not know much about it, which puts the power in the hands of the people you are entrusting. That is a lot of power, as the very essence of your being will be cracked wide open. You will be baring your soul to the unknown. The shaman, and sacred space you are sharing with others and how you share it is a crucial part of this process. Trust and safety are your most important allies in this process. Having as much knowledge about this process will not only help you feel safer, it will give you back your power and enable you to ask the right questions and help make the right decisions, which in turn will make your whole experience much better throughout the whole process.

This guidebook was created to make the whole process easier. For thousands of years *La Madre Ayahuasca (The mother, Ayahuasca)* was used in the Peruvian Jungle by people who did not have the toxic diets and lifestyles present in other areas of the world. It is important to approach this process with the honor and respect previous generations have afforded it. Purifying the mind, body, and spirit prior to an Ayahuasca ceremony is essential to having a more joyful and healing experience. This book outlines how to develop a loving relationship between the spirits of the plants used in the brew and ourselves to establish a deeper connection with the divine, which will bring you closer the teachings it has to offer.

The potent brew known as Ayahuasca has been considered a sacred medicine in South America for centuries. It is grown in the jungle of the Amazon, where the Indigenous Peoples have used it to heal and connect to the human collective and the cosmos. The traditional base ingredients of Ayahuasca are made from a combination of two plants; the Ayahuasca vine *(also known as Vine of the Spirit)* and *Chacruna* leaves, which are native to the rainforests of the Amazon. This combination of plants activates the hallucinogenic DMT *(N, N-Dimethyltryptamine)*. There are also a number of other additive plants, which may be added to the brew depending on the shaman who makes it, according to what his/her intentions are for the healing process.

Ayahuasca is known not only for its unique psychedelic effects, but also for its ability to heal, cleanse, and enlighten. The Indigenous Peoples of the South American tribes have used the healing medicine for centuries to cleanse negative energy while uniting them with the divine. Ayahuasca offers an illuminating pathway, answering many of life's questions. The healing and transformative powers of Ayahuasca have circumnavigated the globe and Ayahuasca tourism has exploded with healing centers popping up in South America and worldwide.

If you have heard the call of the ancient and sacred spirit vine of the Amazon rainforest and can feel her pull, all that is left is to follow in faith. If a trip to South America is financially out of your reach, open your eyes and seek the opportunity to find her spirit presence where you are. When your time arrives, follow her call; do not let your time escape you. She is calling many to herself to ensure the evolution and development of human kind. Many of us are now awakening with a deep yearning to escape our modern lethal lifestyles, which can entangle us. We are searching for more substance and meaning in our lives, which has been stripped away by modern society and keeps us separate from that which is sacred. There are many people who are feeling called to return to nature— and to our true selves.

Ayahuasca provides a bridge for humanity to evolve and raise our consciousness. She will help you understand what is really important in your life and how to be a better person. She enables you to clearly see your weaknesses and strengths. shaman believe that every illness and disease manifests itself energetically first from our thoughts, diet, and lifestyle choices long before it reaches our physical body. Ayahuasca has the ability to cleanse and release these toxic energies. Doors are opened within ourselves, which lead to unknown regions of healing and wisdom. Like a mirror, she reflects back to us our *true* selves and the root causes of our suffering from the deepest regions of our subconsciousness.

We all have the unique opportunity to deepen our connection with all that is and ever was in a sacred ancient place where miracles are born and wisdom is given freely. When you are ready there is no moment as great as the present. Follow your instincts; listen to the signs and take the plunge because *no one is called to Ayahuasca accidentally.*

My Journey

In the summer of 1995 after a series of life-threatening hardships, I met a shaman during a road trip through South Dakota who changed the course of my life. The first thing I noticed about him was the energy surrounding him. It felt charged and surreal as if I was in a dream. He pulled me aside, to the back of his crystal shop, and told me things about my life— details about things he had no way of knowing. He went on to explain some of my past lives and who I really am. He took my hand and told me, *"The path of a healer is never easy."* For the first time in this life it felt someone really saw me. Everything finally made sense.

A decade later, a friend invited me to move to San Francisco where I then became increasingly physically sick. I could not function or think clearly any longer. I went to a variety of doctors who did many tests. To my surprise, these doctors told me I was fine. But I knew better, something was very wrong, so I sought out other avenues of healing.

Remembering how the shaman in South Dakota helped me, I searched for a shaman in the Bay Area. The one I found was trained in Peru to give Ayahuasca ceremonies and invited me to a weekend retreat. It was a powerful and beautiful experience. Things shifted visibly in every aspect of my life after each ceremony. Although I was not healed immediately (from what I later learned was Chronic Lyme Disease), I was healed from some of my symptoms and profoundly healed in other unexpected ways. I was liberated from the depression, which had overwhelmed me from years of the chronic pain brought on from the Lyme Disease as well as from the C-PTSD (Complex Post Traumatic Stress Disorder) symptoms I struggled with. I was also able to see much more clearly about many things, which previously confused me. My energetic vibration increased tremendously, which completely uplifted me in many ways from the wisdom and teachings it brought me.

However, after that experience, my symptoms slowly returned, which I believe was because the shaman I worked did not have enough training. So, I continued my search for healing with a shaman who had more training. At this point I had Chronic Lyme Disease for eight years and it had progressed in my body to a point where I was in pain all the time. I had a very difficult time working or doing much of anything. I lay on the couch like a zombie for years unable to function or have any kind of social life. I felt overwhelmed often; most times I could only stare off into space or meditate for hours seeking some sort of peace and sanity from the mysterious never-ending pain in my body from which no pill or drug could relieve.

Then, one day after doing a powerful visualization practice in a Kundalini Yoga class to break through blockages, which held me back, I visualized myself going to Peru to be healed. Miraculously, only days later a healing Ayahuasca retreat in the Sacred Valley of Peru contacted me and asked me to do a work trade with them. I agreed to do their website and advertising in exchange to be, hopefully, healed from my Lyme symptoms. When I finally arrived at the retreat a week later, I was unfortunately attacked by a dog and had to be stitched up and put on antibiotics. As a result, I was actually healed in the traditional way where only the shaman drank Ayahuasca.

The Shipibo shaman I worked with, Diego Sanchez Rojas, also prescribed a daily plant *Dieta*, which consisted of three plants he kindly brought back for me from the Amazon jungle; *boahuasca, ajos kiros,* and *chuchawasi.* After three ceremonies, all my pain was gone. After eight ceremonies and a powerful Toad Medicine Ceremony *(5meo-dmt),* I was completely healed of all the Lyme symptoms I had suffered with for years and I have only been getting stronger on multiple levels, ever since.

Disclaimer

The information provided in this book is designed to provide helpful information on the subjects discussed through actual findings and in-depth personal research. This book is not meant to diagnose or treat any medical condition.

For diagnosis or treatment of any medical problem, consult with your physician. The publisher and author are not responsible for any specific health needs that may require medical supervision and are not liable for any damages or negative consequences from any treatment, action, application, or preparation to any person reading or following the information in this book.

Chapter 1

The Ayahausca Sacred *Dieta* Protocol

"Your body is a temple, but only if you treat it as one."

— Astrid Alauda

Ayahuasca works to cleanse your body before you can receive beautiful enlightening teachings and experiences. It is beneficial to do some detox cleanses (juice detox or colon detox cleanses etc.) weeks prior to a ceremony to get your body as clean as possible. It is very important to stick to these food and prescription precautions and restrictions prior to a ceremony; not only will it make your experience much more pleasant, but it could save your life.

If you normally have an unhealthy diet, it would be even more crucial for you to focus on cleansing your body at least a month prior to your ceremony to avoid extreme purging; which can show up in a variety of unpleasant ways— physically and energetically— during your ceremony and who wants that?

The Sacred *Dieta* Protocol Weekly Countdown

Eight weeks or more before ceremony, refrain from:

- **SSRI Antidepressants: (Selective serotonin reuptake inhibitors)** *Celexa, Lexapro, Luvox, Paxil, Prozac, Symbyax olanzapine (Zyprexa). Aripiprazole (Abilify), quetiapine (Seroquel), Brexpiprazole (Rexulti), Vilazodone (Viibryd), Vortioxetine (Trintellix* - formerly called *Brintellix).*

- **Benzodiazepines (benzos);** *Alprazolam (Xanax, Xanax XR) Clobazam (Onfi) Clonazepam (Klonopin) Clorazepate*

(Tranxene) Chlordiazepoxide (Librium) Diazepam (Valium, Diastat Acudial, (Diastat) Lorazepam (Ativan).

If you have been taking 'benzos' daily for 6 months or longer:

- Taper off these VERY slowly to avoid serious anxiety and horrifying withdrawal symptoms. This is the proper way, I have found through personal experience and much research, to go off these medications. Cut back 0.25 mg every two weeks. In the last week, take the last 0.25 mg every other day for four days before stopping completely. They can stay in your system for up to **two weeks** after finishing your last dose.

After your last benzo dose, wait another two weeks before doing Ayahuasca. Your nervous system will be extremely sensitive, and you will become more anxious for weeks after your last dose while your body tries to operate on its own again. This medication literally takes over your parasympathetic system, which then relies on the medication to calm down the nervous system, by cutting off the connection to the receptors your body once naturally used to operate on its own.

Do not trust the information on the internet or most retreats about this medication. I have personally gone through this myself. After being on a small dose of *Klonopin* daily for 3+ years, it took me months to ween off properly without having seizures and horrible anxiety.

If you have been on these medications for more than 10 years, it is recommended you cut back only ten percent per month. If you follow this method in weaning off your medications, you will avoid the boomerang effect they create for your nervous system.

Always consult with your doctor about if you should do this and how to accomplish it safely.

Six weeks before ceremony, refrain from:

- MAOI's
- SNRIs, SARIs, NRIs, NDRIs, TCAs, TeCAs and NaSSAs,
- Any other anti-depressants or prescription medications
  Consult with your doctor about if you should do this, and how to do this properly beforehand, as you most likely will have to wean off slowly.
- Recreational drugs (including marijuana)

Four weeks before ceremony, refrain from:

- Benzodiazepines— (if taken just once in a while)
- Sleep medications, including barbiturates
- Processed and canned foods
- All oils and fats
- Fried foods
- Red meat
- Alcohol
- Processed sugars and artificial sweeteners
- Pork
- Duck

Two weeks before ceremony, refrain from:

- Start weaning off caffeine slowly two weeks prior to the ceremony including coffee and black, or green tea, etc.
  This process takes at least two weeks to avoid headaches and other nauseating detox symptoms. Trust me; it is no fun to deal with detox symptoms on top of what you may go through in ceremony.

- Beta blockers, alpha blockers, mixed alpha and beta blockers, calcium channel blockers, ACE inhibitors, angiotensin II receptor antagonists. *Consult with your doctor about if you should do this and how to accomplish it safely.*

- Chocolate– (in large quantities) The *theobromine* in chocolate can cause a fast heartbeat.

- Dairy

- Aged/ smoked foods

- Salt, pepper, spices

- Chilies or other hot peppers

- Ginger, ginseng, nutmeg

- St. John's wort

- Lysergic acid amide (LSA) found in Morning Glory and Baby Hawaiian Woodrose seeds, MDA related herbs (nutmeg, sweet flag).

One week before ceremony, refrain from:

- All caffeine, including coffee, black or green tea, etc.
  This is the final week before going cold turkey! Take your time by slowly cutting back the week prior to avoid headaches and other nauseating detox symptoms.

- Foods containing *Tyramines (see list below)

- Sex (including masturbation)

- Cocaine

- Kratom

- Kava

- Mescaline (any *phenethylamine*)

- Nutritional supplements (e.g., protein powders, herbal remedies, dietary supplements)

- Watching or reading any violent or disturbing movies, news, video games, etc.

72 hours before and after ceremony, refrain from everything already listed, plus:

- Citrus (e.g., lime, lemon, orange)
- Fibrous fruits (e.g., mango, pineapple)
- All caffeine, including coffee, black or green tea, etc. Take at least two weeks to wean off caffeine before quitting today. This way you will avoid unnecessary, excruciating detox symptoms during your ceremony.
- Tomatoes
- Bread

48 hours before a ceremony refrain from everything already listed, plus:

- Betel
- Boswellia
- Carrot seed
- Chamomile
- Cowage
- Curcumin
- Dill seed
- Ephedra
- Fennel seed
- Fo-Ti
- Ginseng
- Horny goat weed

- Kanna
- Kava
- Licorice root
- Parsley seed
- Rhodiola rosea
- Scotch broom
- Siberian ginseng
- Sinicuichi
- Turmeric
- Yerba mate
- Yohimbe

At this point you are certainly asking yourself, what CAN you eat?

Traditionally, the shaman in the Amazon lived on a very bland diet of yucca, plantains, and fish (which have no teeth), rice, avocados, and eggs during their Ayahuasca ceremonies. To stay as clean and safe as possible during your ceremony, these are the foods recommended during the last forty-eight hours prior or you can choose to fast during this time.

- Eggs (hard boiled eggs are best or those cooked without oil, salt, or seasoning)
- Salads greens (freshly squeezed lemon juice works great as a dressing)
- Fresh vegetables
- Fresh fruit (in moderation)
- Sardines or fish without teeth (fresh, not canned)
- Avocados (only freshly ripe, not aged)
- Potatoes

- Rice
- Plantains
- Yucca

Day of ceremony:

- Fast on this day or do not eat anything at least 4 hours prior to drinking Ayahuasca.

One hour before ceremony through to the end of the ceremony, refrain from:

- All fluids should be avoided in the hour leading up to the ceremony, including water (it will make you purge).
  It can be beneficial for you to drink certain herbal teas exactly one hour before drinking Ayahuasca (see *Supportive Plants* chapter).

*Tyramines

It is important to stay away from foods and beverages containing tyramines at least a week prior to ceremony. It will not kill you, but they can make you very sick with a severe headache, which can last for days. They will also accelerate your heartbeat, putting extra pressure on the heart.

Specific foods high in tyramine:

- Figs
- Beer
- Wines
- Walnuts
- Peanuts (in large quantities)
- Brazil nuts (in large quantities)

- Raspberries (in large quantities)
- Fava or broad beans (in large quantities)
- Meat prepared with tenderizers
- Aged cheeses like cheddar, swiss, and blue cheese
- Cured or smoked meats and fish (e.g., sausage, salami, anchovies)
- Over-ripe foods such as bananas, prunes, raisins, or avocados
- Soy products (e.g., soy sauce, teriyaki sauce, miso soup, bean curd, or tofu)
  There have been a number of reported cases directly linking negative effects from combining Ayahuasca with soy products.
- Bouillon-based sauces, shrimp or fish paste/sauces
- Pickled products (e.g., sauerkraut, kimchee, caviar, olives, pickles, etc.)
- Stored foods or spoiled foods
  Only eat fresh food.
- Any food with the word *hydrolyzed* or *autolyzed* in the ingredient list
- Artificial sweeteners (e.g., *Aspartame, NutraSweet*)
- Monosodium glutamate (MSG) or anything with the word *hydrolyzed* which is really MSG
- Coconut and coconut oil (in large quantities)
- New Zealand or hot weather spinach—*tetragonia tetragonioides*, a different plant from regular spinach, *spinacia oleracea*, which is safe (in large quantities)
- Parsley (in large quantities)
- Dill weed (in large quantities)
- Dried seaweed (in large quantities)

- Kombucha (in large quantities)
- Dark chocolate (in large quantities)
  The *theobromine* in chocolate can cause a fast heartbeat.
- Protein extracts
- Liquid or powdered protein dietary supplements
- Canned soups and soups made with protein extracts or bouillon
- Gravies and foods made with meat extracts
- Dried egg whites
- Defatted peanut flour
- Brewer's yeast, yeast vitamin supplements, yeast extracts, foods with yeast ingredients (e.g., Marmite)
- Sourdough bread

Post-Ayahuasca *Dieta*

Follow the Sacred *Dieta* Protocol as outlined in the last seventy-two-hour period for at least three days after your last Ayahuasca ceremony in order to fully integrate your experience.

If you dive back into your old habits too quickly, you do not give your spiritual and energetic body a chance to mend or permit you to feel or see what has shifted. It is more beneficial to continue to follow through this healing process to the very end. After at least three days, then start introducing foods (ideally dates, fruits, root vegetables to ground yourself, and other vegetables- especially greens) and beverages back into your diet slowly. Be gentle with yourself.

Anti-Malaria Medication

Avoid all anti-malaria medications as they interact badly with Ayahuasca. Take precautions for bugs in the retreat you are attending by staying inside as much as possible, especially during sunset and dawn hours. Wear light colored clothing with long sleeves and pants. Use a natural bug spray if possible.

Sexual Restriction

Refrain from sexual activities for a least a week prior to an Ayahuasca Ceremony. The longer you refrain, the better your Ayahuasca experience will be.

The reason: we all have a reservoir of *chi energy*, which we strengthen when we abstain from sex (including masturbation or exchange of any bodily fluids). Chi energy helps the plants teach, guide, and heal us. It has been common practice for thousands of years in various spiritual practices to abstain from any sexual activity in order to strengthen chi energy thus maintaining a stronger connection to the higher frequencies of the divine.

Health Conditions

If you have a weak heart or fragile blood vessels, this will put you at a risk during an Ayahuasca ceremony because of the heavy vomiting it may induce. It also adds stress to the heart from the accelerated heartbeat it brings on. Conditions such as certain eye issues, diabetes, heart disease, and high blood pressure should be discussed in detail with the retreat and your doctor, prior to committing to any ceremony. *You might consider getting an EKG prior to a ceremony if you are unsure of the condition of your heart.*

Chapter 2

Preparing for a Ceremony

"Nearly all men can stand adversity, but if you want to test a man's character, give him power."

— Abraham Lincoln

Choosing a Shaman

During a ceremony you are completely open and vulnerable to all kinds of predatory energies from which only a properly trained shaman can protect you. The shaman you choose for your Ayahuasca ceremony is one of the most important decisions you can make.

Some may think, "the medicine does all the work; it is not a big deal which shaman leads the ceremony" or, "I can do this on my own; who needs a shaman?" But until you have a ceremony take a turn for the worse, either on your own or with a shaman who did not have the right intentions or enough training, you will quickly see how detrimental it is not be guided by a well-trained shaman. In Peru, they say it takes ten years for a shaman to have sufficient training to lead ceremonies properly.

Shaman are responsible for containing the proper space in a ceremony for your protection and for guiding the energies within the space. They should make you feel safe— no question should be in your mind regarding your safety. Doing Ayahuasca without a proper shaman (or a shaman who does not have a clear intention) guiding you or within an improper setting will diminish the power of the healing as at best or diminish your safety at worst.

Establishing trust with a shaman in this delicate environment is very important for your healing process. Each ceremony can be very different depending upon the shaman leading it. Each shaman adds their own flavor; they can play a large part in how your journey will go. Who they are, how much training they have, and their intention for you, affects the outcome for your healing.

You do not want to end up regretting a ceremony when it can easily be avoided. Guiding you through what to watch out for in the beginning can make the difference between being powerfully healed in a beautiful transformative way or being emotionally and mentally traumatized, making it difficult to ever trust another shaman or wanting to experience the medicine ever again.

It breaks my heart when I hear stories from people who had a bad experience with the medicine in this way. Instead of the medicine bringing them to a higher vibration of healing and opening their lives to the highest potential possible, they are scared away never to touch the medicine again. When an Ayahuasca ceremony is performed properly with the right shaman, its transformational healing powers are astounding. It can allow you to achieve the joy, happiness, and prosperity you were put on this Earth to receive.

What to expect from a Shaman

Shaman have historically worked as a guide between worlds; a hollow reed from which spirits can work through to help others. So, it is not the shaman who does the actual healing; he is only a guide or director for the healing spirits and energies. The best shaman are like project managers who make contracts with their personal healing doctor spirits and your spirit guides— to heal you and make you stronger.

An authentic shaman spends many years developing close relationships with various healing plants from the Amazon Jungle by doing plant *dietas*. In this way, they develop a relationship with the healing doctor spirits each brings, who are in animal and/or human form. After years of discipline and devotion, shaman gain respect and protection from these spirits so they can in turn heal you. They can also easily lose the respect and guidance from those helping spirits if they abuse their power; letting ego, greed, and other self-serving behaviors take over.

Ideally, the shaman should also help you process and integrate your experience (or have others around who can) after the ceremony; allowing you to gain further clarity and insight from your journey. An authentic shaman can see your energy field much more clearly in a ceremony through the plant medicine Ayahuasca and can share with you some feedback on what blocks or illnesses they saw.

Ask

When choosing a shaman for your ceremony, *never be afraid to ask* about the training and history of the shaman who will be leading the ceremony. Do not blindly trust a resort or shaman because of an appearance of authenticity or good reviews on a website. The best way to feel confident about your decision is to ask others (if you are a woman, be sure to ask other women) who have had a ceremony with them in the past to determine what their experience had been like.

Shaman from Ecuador

It is important to note that in Ecuador, shaman are regulated. They must meet high standards of training and qualifications in order to lead ceremonies. So, you know when you are attending a ceremony in Ecuador, that the shaman has the appropriate training to work with the medicine in a positive way to protect you. Whereas in Peru, there are no guidelines, and anyone can call himself or herself a shaman and lead an Ayahuasca ceremony, regardless of training.

Discipline

The longer a shaman has dieted, not only with Ayahuasca but other plants of the jungle, shows their commitment and devotion to healing, as well as well as their selflessness and discipline regarding your healing and their overall spiritual strength as a healer. Plant *dietas* are not easy and require a person to have much dedication to their path. Also, shaman who have dieted with many plants have a much deeper connection with many different kinds of energies and doctor spirits, which in turn help you heal in deeper ways.

If the shaman you are working with has only worked with Ayahuasca, they will not have the protection and strength the other plants in *Dieta* would have given them, therefore they have fewer 'tools' in their healing toolbox with which to work. Throughout history, Ayahuasca has been used in a shaman's training alongside other healing spirit plants from the jungle to heal in a powerful synergistic way.

The Inner Circle

If you can, meet the shaman in person. Talk to them, see how they live, pay attention to what kind of people are in their inner circle and, most importantly, listen to your gut instinct. If dysfunctional relationships surround them, this is a sign they have not done enough of their own shadow work. The energies they are attracting into their inner circle are a mirror to their values and morals. They may say their intention is for your higher good, but it is best to watch how they treat you and others— actions speak much louder than words.

Brujos

Brujos are shaman sorcerers who do not work with the light. They do not have your best interest in mind and are notoriously narcissistic. Since they are coming from a place of inner depletion, they are known to be greedy for attention, money, and power.

They are also likely to be controlling of others around them. Some form of dishonesty will be visible in their words or actions. They will have an air about them that they are better than you and will try to disempower you in some way. **It should never be about them.** It is always about you and your healing process. *Brujos* can also steal your energy during a ceremony, which will make you feel sick and drained the next day.

Some *brujos* may be obvious, others are not at first. They may even come across as sincere, charming, caring, and capable. However, at some point their mask, or persona, will slip away. Their dishonesty will be revealed in their words or actions. Disharmony will surround them in some way. You may feel off or uncomfortable in their presence. They may not make you feel completely safe. Eventually in time, shaman who are not coming from a good place will be unveiled.

Shaman of the Light

Nobody is all light or all dark and it is said the best of shaman walk the middle path. However, there are shaman who work more consciously through the selfless force of love, and therefore have a greater capacity to channel light, wisdom, and joy into your healing experience. These shaman can be easily recognized by the love they exude as they walk the path of heart. I was told once you could tell how much goodness a shaman has by how much he or she smiles. Laughter and humor come from the heart— a place of joyful, unburdened spirituality.

A good shaman is selfless and compassionate toward others. The path of a shaman is normally one of 'the wounded healer.' The most authentic of shaman have lived very hard lives themselves, filled with difficult struggles or a near death experience. Those who have lived through the darkest regions of suffering and found the strength to heal themselves and then others are among the most gifted of shaman.

Who is better equipped to help others than someone who has been in the trenches themselves?

Also, money is not an issue for the most spiritually ethical shaman. They usually help those in financial need with a sliding scale or some small exchange of what you can give. There is much controversy around healers and money. Personally, I feel authentic healers who are truly working from their heart have a special kind of awareness and connection to the spiritual realms where material things do not matter so much. Healing becomes tainted when it comes from a place of greed, available only for the rich. Shaman who work with the powerfully healing force of love can see beyond ego and the illusions of the material world.

You should feel good in the presence of the shaman you are entrusting to crack your soul/energetic field wide open. This is no small matter. Pay close attention to how you feel after you leave them. If you feel drained or anything questionable, something is not right. You should feel like you have more energy, are uplifted, see things with more clarity, and feel cleansed for hours or days after being with them. You should feel drawn towards them and want to be around them.

Green Shaman

Green shaman are those who have not trained long enough, and therefore not fully competent to lead ceremonies. In this case, it would be ethical for them to be upfront and honest with you about this and charge you less for their ceremonies until they are more skilled. At this beginning stage, they most likely have not done enough shadow work to discover who they truly are.

Shaman need to do a lot of shadow work and conduct many ceremonies in order to heal their own 'stuff' before they can be available enough to help you. Their own issues will get in the way of your healing process.

I have seen shaman who started out with the best intentions, turn into *brujos* once their facades fall away and they start to obtain power. How a person deals with money and power will clearly reveal their true essence over time.

If you decide to take a chance and do a ceremony with a green shaman it may not be a bad thing, but this is very delicate ground. Any doubts or mistrust you may have with the shaman leading your ceremony could lead to a damaging experience. Trust and safety are always most important. I would suggest you take your time to meditate and pray for guidance in this situation, listen carefully to others who have sat with them previously, and follow your gut feelings.

Peruvian Shamanic History

In Peru, Ayahuasca has been a sacred plant for centuries. Only master (*maestro*) shaman, who have trained for at least ten years were qualified enough to lead Ayahuasca ceremonies. They do extensive *dietas*, not only with Ayahuasca, but other plants in the Amazon. They strive to develop a deep relationship with these plants in a disciplined way in order to connect with the doctor spirits of these plants, who then in turn work with the shaman to heal the local people in their area.

They begin this training from a very young age and are normally 'chosen' by a family member who has also worked with the medicine themselves for most of their lives. This is how it has always been; a long lineage of shaman dating back thousands of years. However, times have changed. Now, most of the younger generation are no longer interested in pursuing this disciplined way of life and are seduced by material things; toxic partying, technology, and fast food that has been inching its way into the deepest regions of the jungle.

At the time of this printing, the average person in Peru makes only thirty-five *soles* per day, while the average shaman charges from 350 to 600 *soles* per person for each ceremony, which are usually groups of ten to thirty people. Not surprisingly, shaman are coming out of the woodwork, many of whom have little experience with the medicine. Many of these shaman are being seduced and corrupted by money and power, often taking advantage of the countless wide-eyed and naive tourists who are increasingly flooding South America each year. Some are very sick people seeking true healing and luckily some will find it. Hopefully the rest will read this book!

Shaman who once worked with integrity, humbleness, and pure devoted love for their family and local villagers, are now finding themselves being forced into living a capitalist way of life. Some quickly learn that in order to thrive as a shaman in this new paradigm they must offer the most powerful ceremonies; often brewed with the highest amount of DMT and other admixtures with the most 'fireworks' for which these seekers are often looking. They end up forsaking the much-needed fragile care and integration most Westerners need to process this new higher vibrational energy.

What ends up happening is that most shaman start out with the best intentions but turn dark once captivated by these powers, which are still relatively new to their culture. There are even highly sought after 'rock star shaman' who have devoted groupies worshipping them as well as sending others their way. This in turn can inflate a shaman's ego to an unhealthy high.

It is easy to understand how people can get caught up in this new lifestyle, especially in a culture that has more than its fair share of poverty. Historically, money, power, and spirituality have never mixed well. This can result in a variety of consequences, some good, but most bad. It is important is to know what to watch out for and how to protect yourself in this transitionally challenged movement.

Choosing a Retreat

Proceed with caution when choosing a healing retreat. There has been a lot of money pouring into South America over the last decade with seekers wanting to heal or experience Ayahuasca and other healing medicines. The amount of money a healing retreat can generate has never before been seen in these parts of the world.

Unfortunately, there are many business-minded people who do not have your best interest at heart and take advantage of the sick and suffering. This has created an imbalance with the spiritual aspect of Ayahuasca. Traditionally, it was used without any money exchanged and only the shaman drank the medicine to heal their village people.

Now, shaman are moving away from their villages and their families. Retreat positions are also being filled with those who want to become shaman but have inadequate training. In worst case scenarios, there may be a *brujo* working at the retreat. You are opening yourself up in a big way spiritually and energetically and greed can taint your experience in so many ways It will affect the healing you receive with this powerful plant medicine.

Make sure to do thorough research before choosing a retreat center. Just because a healing center comes up at the top of a Google search and has a pretty website does not mean it will be good for you. In fact, these centers can be the priciest and the least authentic. More often than not the shaman and workers are overworked and underpaid, which may make guests leave feeling unsatisfied.

Also, some of these centers hold ceremonies with more than twenty people in a group, trying to make as much money as they can, which further diminishes the intimacy of your experience and your healing. The smaller the retreat, the more attention you will receive from the shaman and the deeper the bonds you will form with the other participants in the group.

People tend to think if something costs more, it must be better. Right? Wrong! Remember the dollar goes a long way in South America, so be sure wherever you are going your money is spent well.

You can search using websites such as ayaadvisor.org or reddit.com to find reviews for Ayahuasca centers. However, I have found these reviews are not always a completely accurate reflection of a retreat center. The center may have changed dramatically since the reviews were written or they may have completely different owners and staff with different shaman preforming the ceremonies by the time you show up. I also have heard of people who are given gifts or discounts to leave good reviews. False reviews by the retreats marketing team have also been posted.

I found most people who have had a bad experience are often reluctant to leave a bad review out of fear. They may have been tricked into feeling it is their fault something bad happened when it was not their fault at all. This is a tricky business. If you do not know how things should be run at a healing center or how the facilitators and shaman should treat you, you can easily be manipulated into thinking it is you, not them.

It is good to keep an open mind and find what will work for you. Just because one center did or did not work for one person does not mean the same will be true for you. It all depends on the experience you hope to have and what you want to get out of it. Some people prefer to have an authentic experience, while others prefer to have all the comforts and amenities available to them.

So, how can you really know?

- Listen to your gut.
- Listen to your heart.
- Do your own research.

Try to find people who have most recently been to a retreat you are interested in and ask them how about their experience. If you are currently in the area, ask around. If you are not in the area, go on Facebook and look up spiritual/Ayahuasca/plant medicine related groups in The Sacred Valley or in the Amazon Jungle near Iquitos, Peru and post questions about which centers they recommend. You can also find Ayahuasca forums online to join and talk to people who have been to several different centers.

Sacred Medicine Smorgasbord

Be wary of retreats who try to lure you in by offering many kinds of healing medicines from the shaman smorgasbord; *Kambo* (frog medicine), *bufo alvarius* (5-meo-dmt, toad medicine*), san pedro* (cactus/mescaline*), psilocybin* (mushrooms) in a short amount of time without proper diagnosis or evaluation of your state of mind.

Mixing other sacred medicines along with Ayahuasca within a week or two can be too much, even dangerous. Most people's nervous systems and psyches cannot take all the energy these medicines break open within. Each one of these medicines is very powerful on it is own. Throughout history, up until this point, they were never taken in succession in such short periods of time.

Mixing *bufo alvarius* or using any synthetic form of *5-meo-dmt* shortly after Ayahuasca; which contains *B. caapi*, an MAO inhibitor; can be extremely dangerous. You must be careful there is no MAO-I in the bloodstream before taking the toad medicine. I have read some retreats offer *bufo alvarius* within six to ten hours after an Ayahuasca ceremony. It was also noted that their Aya brew only has *chacruna* added and nothing else.

I have also heard of people having problems, sometimes lasting for years, after doing *psilocybin)* shortly after an *Ayahuasca* or 5-meo-dmt experiences. 5-meo-dmt is very potent on its own and it changes the experiences of all other sacred medicines done afterward to match the 5-meo-dmt experience y creating 're-activations.' This means your experience on these other medicines will largely by influenced by 5-meo-dmt making you feel like you are just doing some warped form of toad medicine.

On psychedelic integration forums, I have read some horror stories of people having full-blown psychotic episodes and not being able to function in their lives for months or years after experiencing too many sacred medicines in a short period of time. Some of these people had put in a great deal of spiritual preparation and they thought they were ready. It is important that you pace yourself and give respect to each of these medicines and the power each has. Each medicine should be fully integrated before moving on to the next. You must pay attention to what is going on for you inside before embarking on a journey with another sacred medicine.

Less can definitely be more. Even if you have to step away from a ceremony to process what happened the night before. Do not be afraid to ask to take a step back in order to rest to take care of yourself. Always do what feels right for you. This can be a little tricky— as it is best to distinguish if this is coming from a place of fear or from knowing that you really need a break. Meditate on it and get in touch with your quiet inner voice.

Ayahuasca can work well with another medicine such as *san pedro* after your ceremonies as it is very grounding and therefore helps the un-grounded feeling you can get from Ayahuasca. *Kambo* can be good to work with before an Ayahuasca ceremony for cleansing, but only if you are with a trained shaman who can diagnose you first and let you know if these things will be good for you personally.

If a retreat offers sacred medicines and charges you beforehand with no opportunity for a refund before you are diagnosed to do these medicines, it is a clear indicator they are only seeking profit and not looking out for your well-being.

Chapter 3

The Spiritual *Dieta*

"Flower will not grow, if the stem does not allow"

— Nayreil

The Ayahuasca *Dieta* is not only about what you eat— it includes what you read, what you watch, and what you listen to. It is your surroundings, the people you choose to hang out with, and the people you are intimate with. Be especially mindful of what you put into your body— emotionally, spiritually, and physically— in the weeks leading up to your Ayahuasca ceremony.

During a ceremony, the most recent things you have fed your body physically, consciously, spiritually; including everything and everyone you are surrounded with in all ways will show up in the forefront of your subconsciousness. Your diet and most recent thoughts will impact your experience in a negative way if you are not careful. I have been in ceremonies where individuals had watched horror movies or violent videos right before a ceremony— eek! These images and the feelings they provoke will most likely show up in your ceremony.

For example, one of the guests of a retreat I was attending had watched some horror movie right before a ceremony. During his ceremony one of the facilitators was fanning him with a large feather and sage to protect him and dispel negative energy. The guest thought it was a knife instead of a feather and imagined the facilitator was trying to kill him!

Ayahuasca begins to work with you the moment you decide to do a ceremony. She is listening and you become a sponge absorbing everything around you in the weeks leading up to a ceremony.

Besides sticking to the sacred *Dieta* and cleansing yourself with organic fruits, vegetables, spring water, and juice fasts in the weeks prior to your Ayahuasca ceremony, you should surround yourself with positive things. Read books and watch movies/documentaries focused on enlightenment and self-growth. Spend time in nature and surround yourself with positive people. Take classes such as Bikram yoga or Kundalini yoga, which help strengthen, expand, and clear your energetic field. Receive other energetic and physical healings, such as reiki or therapeutic massages, etc.

Ask to receive help and teachings in a beautiful and gentle way and gain the insight and strength to overcome any obstacles that may arise. Focus on random acts of kindness, helping others as much as you can in healthy ways, with no expectation of receiving in return. Spend time each day in meditation, developing an internal dialog with *Madre Ayahuasca*, giving thanks and gratitude for the opportunity to be a part of the healing not just for yourself, but for the planet in your upcoming ceremony.

The results will guide you to the most beautiful and enlightening ceremony possible. Your intention and devotion, humility and respectfulness, are the most powerful allies you have during any spiritual practice. Everything you fill your mind with and surround yourself with will present in your Ayahuasca ceremony tenfold. It is not a guarantee of no difficulty, but by following this advice, you will definitely help transform your experience into something much gentler and more beautiful.

Recommended Book List

The Way to Love: The Last Meditations of Anthony de Mello
Anthony de Mello

Aya Awakenings: A Shamanic Odyssey
Rak Razam

The Ayahuasca Sessions: Conversations with Amazonian Curanderos and Western Shamans
Rak Razam

The Ayahuasca Test Pilots Handbook: The Essential Guide to Ayahuasca Journeying
Chris Kilham

The Kin of Ata are Waiting for You
Dorothy Bryant

The Four Agreements: A Practical Guide to Personal Freedom, a Toltec Wisdom
Don Miguel Ruiz

Shedding the Layers: How Ayahuasca Saved More than My Skin
Mark Flaherty

Inner Paths to Outer Space: Journeys to Alien Worlds through Psychedelics and Other Spiritual Technologies
Rick Strassman MD, Slawek Wojtowicz, Luis Eduardo Luna, Ede Frecska

The Dream: A Spiritual Journey of Self-Healing
Chris Taylor

The Presence Process: A Journey into Present Moment Awareness
Michael Brown

The Untethered Soul: The Journey Beyond Yourself
Michael A. Singer

John of God: The Brazilian Healer Who's Touched the Lives of Millions
Heather Cumming, Karen Leffler, Goswami Ph.D., Amit

The Wisdom of the Enneagram: The Complete Guide to Psychological and Spiritual Growth for the Nine Personality Types
Don Richard Riso

The Fasting Path: For Spiritual, Emotional, and Physical Healing and Renewal
Stephen Harrod Buhner

Senses of the Soul: Emotional Therapy for Strength, Healing and Guidance
Guru Meher Kahlsa

The Mood Cure: The 4-Step Program to Take Charge of Your Emotions
Julia Ross

The Anti-Anxiety Food Solution
Trudy Scott, James Lake

The Autoimmune Paleo Cookbook: An Allergen-Free Approach to Managing Chronic Illness
Mickey Trescott, Kyle Johnson, Sarah Ballantyne

The Gerson Therapy: The Proven Nutritional Program for Cancer and Other Illnesses
Charlotte Gerson, Morton Walker

The Complete Master Cleanse: A Step-by-Step Guide to Maximizing the Benefits of The Lemonade Diet
Tom Woloshyn

Medical Medium: Secrets Behind Chronic and Mystery Illness and How to Finally Heal
Anthony, William

Discover Your Authentic Self: Be You, Be Free, Be Happy
Sherrie Dillard

Munay-Ki Abundance: Spiritual Journey of a Wisdom Keeper
Malcolm J. Wilkins

Autobiography of a Yogi
Paramahansa Yogananda

The Power of Intention: Learning to Co-create Your World Way
Dr. Wayne W. Dyer

Women of Wisdom
Allione Tsultrim

Feeding Your Demons: (Shadow Work) Ancient Wisdom for Resolving Inner Conflict
Allione Tsultrimn

The Highly Sensitive Person: How to Thrive When the World Overwhelms You
Elaine Aron

Supernatural: Meetings with the Ancient Teachers of Mankind
Graham Hancock

Spiritwalker: Messages from the Future
Hank Wesselman

Visionseeker: Shared Wisdom from the Place of Refuge
Hank Wesselman

Medicinemaker: Mystic Encounters on the shaman's Path
Hank Wesselman

The Seven Spiritual Laws of Success: A Practical Guide to the Fulfillment of Your Dreams
Deepak Chopra

Medicine for the Soul: The Complete Book of Shamanic Healing
Ross Heaven

Cave and Cosmos: Shamanic Encounters with Another Reality
Michael Harner

The Path of the Priestess: Discover Your Divine Purpose
Rose Cole, Jane Ashley, Sofia Thom, Jena La Flamme et al.

Journey of Souls: Case Studies of Life Between Lives
Michael Newton

Compassionate Action
Chatral Rinpoche, Zach Larson

The Yoga Sutras of Patanjali
Alistair Shearer (translator)

The Yogi's Roadmap: Pantanjali Yoga Sutra as a Journey to Self-Realization
Bhavani Silvia Maki, Rama Jyoti Vernon, Mariana Caplan

The Journey Home: Autobiography of an American Swami
Radhanath Swami

Heavenly Streams: Meridian Theory in Nei Gong
Damo Mitchell, Robert Aspell

Siddhartha
Hermann Hesse

When Things Fall Apart: Heart Advice for Difficult Times
Pema Chodron

Shaman, Healer, Sage: How to Heal Yourself and Others with the Energy Medicine of the Americas
Alberto Villoldo

The Power of Now: A Guide to Spiritual Enlightenment
Eckhart Tolle

No Man is an Island
Thomas Merton

The Incredible Life of a Himalayan Yogi: The Times, Teachings and life of Living Shiva: Baba Lokenath Brahmachari
Shuddhaanandaa Brahmachari, Ann Shannon

Mastery of Consciousness: Awaken the Inner Prophet: Liberate yourself with yogic wisdom. Break the limits of mind, body and life circumstances
Nandhi Tapasyogi

Discover Your Psychic Type: Developing and Using Your Natural Intuition
Sherrie Dillard

Black Elk Speaks: Being the Life Story of a Holy Man of the Oglala Sioux
John G. Neihardtm Standing Bear

The Myth of Freedom and the Way of Meditation
Chogyam Trungpa, Pema Chodron

Carlos Castaneda Books:

o The Teachings of Don Juan: A Yaqui Way of Knowledge, 1968

o A Separate Reality: Further Conversations with Don Juan, 1971

o Journey to Ixtlan: The Lessons of Don Juan, 1972

o Tales of Power, 1974

o The Second Ring of Power, 1977

o The Eagle's Gift, 1981

o The Fire from Within, 1984

o The Power of Silence: Further Lessons of Don Juan, 1987

o The Art of Dreaming, 1993

o Magical Passes: The Practical Wisdom of the Shamans of Ancient Mexico, 1998

o The Wheel of Time: Shamans of Ancient Mexico, Their Thoughts About Life, Death and the Universe, 1998

o The Active Side of Infinity, 1999

Recommended Movie List
(Most titles on the Gaia Channel are good to watch)

Song of the New Earth
Ward Serrill

Baraka
Ron Fricke

Samadhi
Daniel Schmidt

Samsara
Ron Fricke

Choice Point
Harry Massey, Myfanwy Marshall

Inner Worlds, Outer Worlds
Daniel Schmidt

DMT: The Spirit Molecule
Mitch Schultz

Peaceful Warrior
Victor Salva

Avatar
James Cameron

Waking Life
Richard Linklater

Tuning In
David Thomas

The Living Matrix
Greg Becker

Sukhavati
Joseph Campbell

Happy
Roko Belic

The Happiness Prescription
Deepak Chopra

I Am
Tom Shadyac

Awake: The Life of Yogananda
Paola di Florio, Lisa Leeman

Healing: Miracles, Mysteries and John of God
John of God, David Unterberg, Andrea Wolffer

Secret of Water
Jirka Rysavy, Saida Medvedeva

K-PAX
Iain Softley

What the Bleep Do We Know?
William Arntz

I Origins
Mike Cahill

I am Not Your Guru
Joe Berlinger

Wake Up
Jonas Elrod, Chloe Crespi

Powder
Victor Salva

Astral City
Wagner de Assis

Healing
Craig Monahan

Heal
Kelly Noonan

Discover the Gift
Demian Lichtenstein, Shajen Joy Aziz

Awake in the Dream
Catharina Roland

Aya Awakenings
Rak Razam

The Last Shaman
Raz Degan

Ayahuasca: Vine of the Soul
Richard Meech

From Neurons to Nirvana: The Great Medicines
Oliver Hockenhul

Recommended Audio Book List
(These titles can be found on Audible.com)

Audio books by Reginald A. Ray

- o *The Practice of Pure Awareness: Somatic Meditation for Touching Infinity*
- o *Awakening the Heart* (Volume 1 & 2)
- o *Your Breathing Body* (Volume 1 & 2)
- o *Somatic Descent*
- o *Meditating with the Body*
- o *Buddhist Tantra*

Feeding Your Demons (Shadow Work): Ancient Wisdom for Resolving Inner Conflict
Allione Tsultrimn

Chapter 4

During the Ceremony

"The real temple is the whole world, and there is nothing as divinely blessed as a blooming growing garden"

— Vera Nazarain

Here are a few suggestions to help make your experience comfortable and safe during your Ayahuasca ceremony.

To begin, make sure you have a thick cushion and blankets. These are normally provided by the retreat, but sometimes are inadequate. Consider bringing extra padding, like a rolled-up inflatable camping cushion or something similar. It is a good idea to have a small folding chair to sit upright as much as possible during your ceremony, as lying down will intensify your experience.

Also, make sure you bring a headlamp with a red light setting, as your eyes will become very light sensitive during a ceremony. You can make one with red tape over a regular headlamp. You may bring sacred stones or ceremonial objects that have meaning for you, which can be placed at the side or foot of your cushion.

It is nice to have a sachet to keep your important items together and will make your ceremony much easier and enjoyable. In doing so, they will not be lost or scattered in the dark. Here are the items I personally like to have on hand: a small bottle of Florida water (you can also keep this in a small spray bottle for spraying on yourself, or into the air surrounding you during ceremony), Palo Santo, white mountain sage, one or two mapacho cigarettes (Peruvian tobacco cigarette) and a lighter. These are all excellent items to have on hand for burning or spraying/applying on yourself during or after ceremony to energetically cleanse your space from negative energies, and/or cover up any unpleasant smells.

Keep your headlamp in the same sachet if you prefer or you can tie it to a strap around your neck or waist with a carabineer clasp that easily opens and closes. This will enable you to pull it off the strap and put it on your head, then put it back on the strap easily if it falls off your head. It is very dark during ceremony and you will most likely feel too disorientated to want to search for it. Even if it is lying by your side you will have a difficult time finding it, especially with other people close by with all their own items.

When the ceremony is over, a thermos with warm peppermint and/or passionflower tea mixed with lemon balm tea is nice to have. Peppermint tea is very soothing and healing for the stomach and throat. Passionflower and lemon balm tea will help calm your mind so you can sleep as your mind will be very active during the ceremony and can stay active for hours afterwards.

Releasing Fear

It is normal to be afraid and feel trepidation rise before a ceremony. A good way to work with releasing fear is by using emotional freedom techniques (EFT) or 'tapping.' Also, a daily practice of Kundalini yoga or Qi Gong is especially helpful as these practices are grounding, strengthen the nervous system, and clear blockages in your energetic body. Practicing Pranayama breathing techniques and learning mantras to focus on before and during ceremony is very helpful. 'Fire of breath' is an especially useful breathing technique that will calm the nervous system down fast!

You can find great videos of these techniques on YouTube. Performing these practices daily for weeks prior to your ceremony is a powerful way of releasing fears by calming down your nervous system, which in turn quiets the mind and emotions.

Fear stems from The ego, which is afraid of change and ego death. Be mindful of letting go of who you believe yourselve to be and what society has taught you to believe. Be open to all possibilities and know that whatever change takes place is ultimately for your higher good.

Keep in mind that we are essentially nothing but pure light and love beneath all the 'static' which has been overlaid upon us over the years of being here on this planet. Focus on that love as a steady candle flame, which is always burning within ourselves and will never be tainted or put out. Energy never dies; it only transforms. Try to stay in your heart and get out of your head. Take a step back from yourself and become a witness to that which will unfold for you.

As long as you prepare properly, according to the guidelines in this book, and work with a good shaman, you will be protected and safe.

Setting an Intention

When you hold up your cup of sacred Ayahuasca brew to your mouth, before you drink, make sure you have given some thought as to what your intention is for the ceremony. What would you like to get out of your ceremony?

An intention is the sincere motivation or question you have for the medicine. Your intention should stem from the deep inner regions of your soul and is paramount for your journey to unfold justly for you in a clear and positive manner. What is the burning question you have deep inside?

If you are unclear, meditate and develop communication with Ayahuasca days or weeks before each ceremony. Remember the ceremony begins the moment you make the decision to journey with her and she is communicating with you from that moment forward.

Make it simple. Do not give her a Christmas list, as she will just give it back to you! On some occasions, she will give you an answer and you may not even realize it until reflecting back on your ceremony months later. Try searching deep within yourself and find exactly what you need. For example, instead of telling the medicine, "I want to quit smoking," ask the medicine to find the root of your addiction and request for strength to help you confront it.

My favorite 'go to' intention is *release that which does not serve me, then gently refill that space with my truth.* This is a powerful intention as we do not always know exactly what it is we need to let go of or what our truth is. Surrender to the wisdom of a higher power.

If you can, read *The Power of Intention* by Wayne W. Dyer. This book is a powerful way to see how our intentions set a clear path in our lives.

After Drinking Ayahuasca

After you drink Ayahuasca and sit down to wait for it to kick in during the quietness. The intense quiet can be a bit unnerving. In traditional ceremonies, the shaman will not sing his *icaros* until later in the ceremony so you may feel a bit of anxiety sitting quietly in the dark waiting for things to happen. I found it is best to focus on mantras or prayers, depending on your religion and what feels comfortable for you.

Personally, mantras work best for me. They are sacred words spoken in *Sanskrit,* which are believed to have special psychological and spiritual powers. Mantra meditation helps induce altered states of consciousness, which can help ease your mind into the Ayahuasca experience with much less trepidation.

Navigating Through Your Visions and Teachings

Resistance

What resists, persists. Be mindful to release expectations of what you hope your ceremony should be like, or what you want it to be like. Trust it is all happening for your higher good, whatever that may be. This is a large part of having a beautiful ceremony. Stay out of your head and go into your heart. Take a step back and get out of your own way. Let yourself be a witness to what is happening without any attachment to it.

Know that any painful past experiences that may come up during the ceremony are for your deepest healing. If you are having a difficult time, remember to breathe. Taking deep breaths will help you stay in touch with your body and get more grounded. Visualize your breath pushing out the unhealthy energies. Trust that any difficult feeling or experience will transform into something beautiful. Let go of thinking any particular experience during the ceremony will last forever. We are fluid and everything changes. Holding on to anything too tightly during ceremony will not serve you; it will only make your experience more difficult. Let it go; let it flow.

Letting go of *resistance* to what is happening is key in your ceremony flowing with ease. As in your ordinary daily life; once you resist, you become stuck, it creates a block, and new energy is not allowed to flow. Make space for the new energy to flow inward. Allow whatever is happening to occur without judgment. If it feels difficult, go into the experience and ask what it has to teach you. Then you can more easily flow through it and move on to the next experience. This is the natural ebb and flow of life, the natural yin and yang of existence. Know there is beauty and bliss waiting for you outside of each painful or difficult experience.

Truth

Have faith your journey will help you access the most healing for your higher good. Each journey you take with Ayahuasca will be completely different. No two experiences will ever be the same. If you have a difficult experience one night, the next night may be blissful beyond your wildest dreams. Why? We are always evolving and changing, so what we need in one moment may not be what we need in the next.

Most of what we have learned in life to this point is not the truth. We should always question everything. It is beneficial to keep an open and flexible mind to other possibilities of what life and truth is for you.

Each of us is essentially made of pure love and awareness. Ayahuasca helps us access this abundant love residing in each one of us by accessing our truth, which shows us our blockages and false beliefs. This ultimately opens our hearts and brings forth the power to heal.

Do not Fight Your Visions

Let your visions and any other sensations move through you, becoming fluid like water. Trust in the higher power of the universe. Understand what is shown to you is for your higher good. Know you will come out of this experience healed and stronger than ever before.

Ayahuasca always gives you what you need, not what you want. Do not try to fight for 'beautiful visions.' If the experience is difficult, breathe through it, focus on your breath. At times, it can raise your vibration by focusing on love— loving thoughts or the love of people or pets in your life. You can pull yourself out of some dark places by tuning into the higher vibration of love. It can change the energy of your experience dramatically.

Have faith in what is happening, as it is exactly what you need in the moment. Nothing is static; the only constant is change. Learning to give up control will serve you greatly both in ceremony as well as in life. Change is inevitable; try to take a step back from yourself and become a witness to what is unfolding. In your ceremony, this is where you will be tested the most. Embracing it will make you much stronger.

Ask

Remember to ask for guidance, wisdom or healing during your ceremony. She is listening. What is the truth for you behind any difficult experience or questions you may have? Ask for teachings for your higher good and she will show you.

Trust

The only way to move past your suffering and disease is to fully trust the process. What you resist, persists. You have to walk through the fire of your inner suffering and feel it fully so you can embrace it, learn from it, and move past it. You need to face the things you do not want to see in order to heal. Once you have a deeper understanding of your life's most painful experiences, you can be set free. The vine of Ayahuasca will caress you with the love of a mother, submerge you in her divine knowledge, taking you by the hand to otherworldly realms of innermost wisdom.

Deep Healing

Try not to go online and focus on other people's experiences. Your experience will be unique to you. Some people will talk about one or two experiences and say it was 'bad' and 'they will never do it again.' It is not always easy to see the darker aspects of ourselves. These people who see it as 'negative' are more than likely not ready to explore or accept negative characteristics about themselves.

It is essential to look at your faults or traumatic memories, which have kept you stuck in unhealthy patterns. These energetic patterns eventually become crystalized in your body, which becomes a breeding ground for physical disease. You need to heal your thinking and behaviors in order to heal deep wounds—as above, so below.

My first four ceremonies were full of beautiful teachings and I did not get physically sick or purge even once. I have heard of others who did up to twenty ceremonies before they purged. Purging is not as bad as we see it in this culture. In the Peruvian culture, purging is viewed as a healthy way for your body to release energetic and emotional energies not serving the body. After purging, everyone feels much lighter and better.

If you are seeking deep healing from a state of bad health, it may take ten to twenty ceremonies to clear out your body, heart, and mind of toxic energetic states before you are healed. Try to not be afraid of going through this process. In the end you will be glad you did. Would you rather spend a lifetime of suffering with an illness or have it healed in a dozen or so ceremonies?

It does help if you have performed several spiritual practices before your ceremonies or have a daily meditation and yogic routine in place. If so, you will most likely go to the lighter side of healing right away. It all depends on how mindful you are in your daily life, how much shadow work you have done for yourself, and how much you can be fluid and understand the energies which present themselves to you.

Be Grateful

Always be grateful for your experiences throughout the ceremony, whether they are difficult or easy. Remember to say, "thank you" for this extraordinary process in which you are taking part. You are having the privilege to communicate directly with the universal consciousness and all the wisdom and healing she can bring to you. That is incredible! How many people have this unique opportunity? Being in a state of gratitude for everything that comes up will help establish the right kind of frequency you need for authentic healing to take place. Being grateful attracts the right kind of energy to help your process.

Healing with Ayahuasca

Ayahuasca is a very powerful healing plant, but it is important to keep in mind that this plant medicine is only one among many. Many people come to experience this plant medicine because of its growing popularity, but it may *not* be the plant you actually need. It is wise to see a shaman who knows and has done a *Dieta* with many plants, so they can give you what you need. Ayahuasca is only one tool in the healing toolbox; it is not a complete solution.

Listen to your heart. Only do Ayahuasca if it calls to you. If you do feel called to Ayahuasca, it requires deep introspective work from your end. During your healing process with Ayahuasca it is best to consciously step outside yourself to look at how you perceive in your life from different perspectives. Ayahuasca mirrors your subconsciousness so you can clearly see your fears and blockages, which are key areas for growth and healing.

Most of us have repressed fears, which can come out distorted. We may misinterpret what is really happening, which is why working with an integrative therapist (who knows the process of entheogens) afterwards is vital for your healing process. Focus on what is coming up for you to heal with an open mind rather than just focusing on the afterglow.

It is also more powerful to have a well-trained shaman prescribe and monitor other plants for you to *Dieta* along with Ayahuasca on your retreat. In this way you can be strengthened, healed, and protected even further in the area you are seeking to heal. These other plant medicines can be integrated into your healing protocol before, during, or after doing an Ayahuasca ceremony retreat.

How Ayahuasca Will Not Heal You

You will only go as far with your healing as you want to go. It takes much discipline and a daily practice of awareness and mindfulness to change years of unhealthy habits, patterns, and beliefs. Ayahuasca is not a magic pill. It will bring you awareness and give you powerful insights of your inner landscape in all kinds of ways, but the real ceremony really begins once you leave the retreat ceremony. *Your daily life will now become the true ceremony.*

The day after your ceremony, write down in detail all the wisdom and visions you received during your ceremony. This will help you process your new awareness. Obstacles and challenges that you may have been repressing or ignoring will begin to show up in your life ten-fold, which will require conscious healing on your part long after the Ayahuasca ceremony is over. Ayahuasca will continue to work in your life to heal you further and make you stronger. It will be your decision to make every choice consciously for your higher good.

Even though it may seem you will never forget what happened in your ceremony, as it is more real than reality, in time you will not clearly remember it all. Most of us live a lifetime avoiding what feels bad and turning towards what feels good. For deep healing to manifest, it is vital to see and feel our wounds fully. We need to fully embrace the greater truth and let go of our attachments in order to truly release our suffering.

The trauma brought into our lives is only how we perceive it. We often only see a small perspective of what really happened. We often misinterpret other people's perspectives because of our limited perspective. We can also become selfish, frigid, or limited in our views of what happened. The lack of self-love and self-absorption, which often occurs when we try to heal our wounds, can perpetuate us into a cycle of being a victim rather than liberating us.

Expansion is key. Keep a daily journal, practice meditating, yoga, breathing techniques, *Thai Chi*, *Qi Gong,* and other spiritual disciplines to help move inner energies and clear blocks within yourself, which will liberate you from disharmony.

During the Retreat

If you are serious about receiving the most healing possible, it is advisable to avoid computers or other distractions such as music, reading, or conversing with others during your Ayahuasca retreat. The most crucial inner work takes place after a ceremony. Tune in to yourself, be mindful to what you are feeling and experiencing, as well as what feelings arise for you towards others in the group including the shaman. It is common for people to direct unhealed energy towards the shaman, which is another good reason to choose a well-trained shaman, as they will know how to handle this and protect themselves.

This becomes very touchy ground because everyone and everything will be a mirror to what is coming up for you. Write it all down and spend your time meditating, journaling, drawing, or painting. Some people struggle with this, especially those who are not used to being alone without distractions or do not have a daily meditation practice.

Most of us are bombarded with constant distractions. However, 'unplugging' from the world and 'plugging' into yourself and to the divine is a very important part of the healing process. It is a time to slow down and go within. Also keep in mind, you cannot always trust your visions during your ceremonies. It is possible that you may be very wrong about what they are really saying to you and they may change their meaning in time. Try not to struggle with deciphering your visions or experiences right away. Just write them down, and let it go. The true meaning will come to you at the right time.

I believe one of the reasons visions may be misleading is we all have the choice to change the path on which we are traveling. Certain visions may be showing you the path for your highest good on your current path. We all have much power and greatness within us to change our minds and the course of our path; we can become almost anything we wish to be.

Take a step back and be a witness to yourself. Watch every choice you make or have made and how every decision you chose played out in your life. This can be a very enlightening experience. The more we are aware of our fears, unconscious behaviors, and patterns the more each of us can step into the light of who we truly are. This can look much different than who we have known ourselves to be.

Many of us have a lot of repressed emotions, feelings, and memories that we have kept hidden for most of our lives. When they come up, it makes sense that they may appear to be confusing or distorted. Take time to process this and keep an open mind during your retreat. Stay open to all possibilities.

Try to stick to the bland *Dieta* and not become frustrated. Some people get angry at the restrictions and leave the retreat feeling they are not getting their money's worth or they feel they are being treated poorly when given only a few simply prepared food choices. The sacred *Dieta* is meant to be bland. The space you are in is meant to be void of any distractions. Both are traditional ways of working with the medicine, as it has been for hundreds of years.

Some retreats may offer more to make the experience more attractive to everyone and enhance personal growth, like attending mindfulness classes about expanding and raising your awareness and consciousness in healthy ways (e.g., planetary awareness, helpful ways of navigating on the medicine, daily yoga classes, painting classes etc.). Each of these can be very helpful for many during this time, to move your energy and focus it in a positive way.

Chapter 5

After the Ceremony

"A person often meets his destiny on the road he took to avoid it."

— *Jean de La Fontaine*

Follow the Post-Ayahuasca *Dieta*

The post-Ayahuasca *Dieta* guidelines are important to follow when you leave the retreat in order to fully integrate the medicine. The medicine will continue to work strongly in your body for days after your last ceremony. It may be very tempting to grab a burger and fries right away but try your best to hold on to the *Sacred Dieta Protocol*, as outlined in the final seventy-two hours, for at least three days after your last ceremony. Also, try to include more root vegetables in your diet at this time to ground yourself as doing multiple Ayahuasca ceremonies can leave you feeling very ungrounded.

If you dive back into your old habits too quickly, it does not give your spiritual and energetic bodies a chance to mend or allow you the chance to feel or see what has shifted. It is more beneficial to continue to follow through with this healing process to the very end. After at least three days, start introducing foods and beverages back into your diet slowly and gently.

I have found that people who attend more ceremonies naturally gravitate towards eating a healthier and cleaner plant based organic food diet because they are vibrating at a higher frequency from all the cleansing healings they received with the medicine. The same thing is true of people who follow a regular yoga practice.

Integration

Integration is the healing which takes place after your ceremonies are over. The healing and teachings you received are now brought into your life where the real work begins. Many things will come up for you which you may not expect. Emotions, which have been suppressed, will continue to pour out and most often are mirrored back to you in your closest relationships.

You may come back to a life you no longer recognize as the same one you left. The veils, which once served you and were held in place in order for you to function in jobs or relationships, are now taken down. Your old beliefs will be shaken and torn apart, ready to be re-built. This can be incredibly freeing, but also difficult as you are now able to see your life much clearer as the truth of who you really are, and what you really value, emerges.

Life is the real ceremony. Your hardest life lessons will now appear magically in front of your eyes, challenging you to approach them differently. In order to fully heal and move on to a healthier and happier being, you will need to recognize how your old patterns no longer serve you. On your own, this often makes life confusing and difficult to manage. It requires much inner strength, insight, mindfulness, and awareness on your part to get through it all. This is all very normal, and part of the healing process.

It is beneficial during this time to find a counselor or life-coach who is familiar in working with people who have used Ayahuasca or other powerful plant medicines. These individuals are skilled in the working with this kind of process and can maximize your healing. The right kind of therapist can help you integrate your teachings and experiences, received while on the medicine, into your life more gracefully and with greater depth. This is especially recommended if you are working through some difficult past traumas, addictions, or other psychological challenges.

This is an empowering and grounding time. You can learn to take life's reigns in your hands. It is the time to let go of playing the victim in your own life. By doing proper shadow work, you will realize you are the only one who can create a happy life for yourself. You are not in control of others or most situations, but you are always in control of how you respond. You can decide to make positive or negative changes in your life when you fully understand the truth of who you are and what you really want in your life; you are deserving of good things.

Shadow Work

Shadow work is one of the most important things to work with after any sacred medicine ceremony to help you see things much more clearly, and to help you through your integration process. Research some good books on shadow work (see the *Recommended Books and Recommended Audio-books* lists in Chapter 3).

Have a Daily Practice

Making time for a daily practice of mindfulness, meditation, or yoga will help you tune in to your feelings and thoughts. Even if you are walking or doing mundane chores throughout the day, pay attention to how you are feeling and what thoughts are presenting themselves to you.

Spend some time in nature. Nature encourages reflection and introspection and is a good way to be in touch with the calming and naturally healing energy of the plants and trees around you. This will clear and strengthen your energetic field, especially in the early weeks after your retreat. Express your gratitude for the healing you have received by doing a simple and effective ancient practice by bringing tobacco (tobacco is a sacred plant in Peru) with you to a special place in nature in and offering it to the earth, saying, "thank you."

Journal your thoughts and feelings before going to bed. Also keep a dream journal to write in as soon as you wake, to record the hidden messages in your dreams that arise from your sub-consciousness while you sleep.

Community

Having a like-minded community to support your journey is vital. After returning home from this amazing life-altering experience, you may find your home is not as you left it. You may try to explain to your family and friends what happened, but you will likely be faced with blank stares, or even worse questions like, "Isn't that just some kind of drug?"

Your life will no longer be the same. If you struggle during this time, it most likely will come from not being able to let go of the things which no longer serve you. Once you can do this, it will become much easier. Only those who have experienced this medicine will be able to fully relate to what you have been through or be prepared for what you will now face. So, to whom do you turn? Do not go through it alone thinking you can be strong enough to face the revelations on your own. Hopefully, you developed some deep connections with those who you did the medicine with or with a therapist who is trained to work with those who have done this kind of medicine. But if not, it is important to search for a spiritual community for support during this time.

Find people who have done the medicine and are as deeply committed to the healing experience as you are. Start a meet-up group if you have trouble finding others. Doing so will help you integrate your experience better and help you grow. Do not take this advice lightly; it can be a daunting matter to deal with the things that will come up.

Things will surface that will confuse you and throw you off track when you least expect it.

As a species, we are 'pack animals.' We are meant to have a tribe to support us, people we can lean on, a team to have our backs. We need people we can relate to and trust. In this day and age there is unrealistic pressure to be strong and independent. Taking the world on our shoulders in this way is a difficult way of life and it is contrary to how we are meant to live. It is built into our DNA. Being alone was a form of punishment long ago; to be cast-off from the 'tribe' was a punishment, which often meant certain death. Being alone subjects us to vulnerabilities. In our minds small things distort to larger things and it is one of the main root causes of mental illnesses and addictions.

Take Care of Your Body

When you are going through a time of stress and difficulty, taking care of your body with simple daily routines makes a big difference in allowing your healing process to go more smoothly. Get out in the sun as much as you can. Try a variety of monthly detox cleanses, fast for a day or longer every week or two. Practice breathing exercises or yoga.

Develop some exercise routine, which will be best for you out in the sun, in nature such as bicycling or hiking. If you work a lot or do not have much time to exercise, try to walk at least twenty to forty minutes each day. Get outside and go for a walk on your work breaks.

Infrared saunas have a wide range of benefits including reducing inflammation and helping both your mind and body detox, it even helps lower your blood pressure (unlike regular saunas). Take up swimming, being in the water is a very healing and a great way to soothe stress and strengthen the body gently. It also improves your balance by working out deep inner balancing muscles required to stay afloat in the water, and it will calm down your nervous system.

If you cannot swim, taking hot baths more regularly will help you feel much better. To make your hot bath more effective, add Epsom salts to each bath along with therapeutic grade essential oils. My favorite is ten to twenty-six drops of peppermint or spearmint oil, which are natural forms of menthol that can help you feel invigorated as well as sooth any aches or pains. There is an ancient Ayurveda essential oil blend, which includes peppermint or spearmint oil (ten to thirty drops) and clove oil (three to five drops), that creates a combination of hot and cold properties that energetically balances out the yin and yang polarities of the body.

Be mindful of your diet. Our bodies, minds, and emotions are made up entirely of what we eat. Stay away from refined sugars and artificial sweeteners. Eat as many fresh organic fruits and vegetables as you can and avoid processed and genetically modified foods. As energetic beings, we take on the energy of the foods we are ingesting. If you are eating foods from plants and animals raised suffering in poor living conditions and fed genetically modified food that has often been sprayed with heavy pesticides and chemicals, you are taking on that negative energy.

It has been proven these foods change your DNA and effect how your digestive system and your mind works. There is an entire eco-system in out guts and unnatural foods and additives throw everything out of balance and create disease.

I personally have found *The Whole 30 Diet* to be the most powerful way to discover which foods strengthens us or weaken us. This is an elimination diet that has helped many of my clients, and me, with chronic pain and inflammation in the body caused by certain foods. Intolerance or allergies to a food are two very different things. Most of us are intolerant to certain foods (usually dairy, soy, grains, legumes and/or processed foods). You can tap into much more energy and strength, release all kinds of pain, emotional problems, migraines, and other health issues if you eliminate certain foods from your diet.

Chapter 6

Supportive Plants

"Nature itself is the best medicine"

— Hippocrates

Lemon Balm (*melissa officinalis)*

Lemon balm inhibits GABA-T transaminase, which allows GABA *(gamma-aminobutyric acid)* to build up in the brain. This works in a unique way with Ayahuasca, as it will help you feel more relaxed, easing you into the experience.

This is also one of the two known plants (the other being passionflower) that can greatly help with nausea and stomach problems that can occur after drinking Ayahuasca. Lemon balm is also known to intensify your visions and make them more colorful than usual.

Timing is very important with this, drinking the lemon balm tea no later than one hour before ingesting Ayahuasca. If you drink this tea any sooner than an hour, it may not kick in at the right time to help your stomach. Remember, you should not drink any fluids in the final hour before drinking Ayahuasca or during the ceremony at all as it will make you purge.

Regardless, drinking lemon balm tea before an Ayahuasca ceremony will always help make your experience a more positive one. I know some will argue the purging is an important part of the cleansing process. Lemon balm will not stop it completely, but it will lessen the intensity and help those who have ongoing stomach problems.

According to traditional herbal medicine, lemon balm is known as the 'great facilitator.' It is shown to improve the effect of all other medicinal herbs with which it is taken. In alchemic legend, lemon balm is the herb *paracelsus* used to make his 'ens' known to be a potent restorative health elixir made from alchemic methods.

Passionflower *(passiflora incarnate)*

Passionflower is known to enhance the effects of other substances, most notably in Ayahuasca or *psilocybin* (mushrooms). This is because the MAOIs in passionflower mimic the same compounds in Ayahuasca, which increases the DMT effects. In some regions of the Amazon, tribal groups add passionflower in the admixture of the Ayahuasca brew for these reasons.

If you drink passionflower as a tea before a ceremony, it is known to prolong the experience and give it a euphoric spin. It can also be smoked at the end of a ceremony to prolong the experience even further. Its sedative properties help with unpleasant effects during a ceremony such as anxiety, restlessness, a racing heart, and headaches. It is also used to prevent seizures and help you sleep better after your ceremony.

Passionflower is the herb used by extraordinary full trance medium healer, John of God in Brazil. He personally blesses and prescribes this herb to all who come to see him or do long distance healings with him because of its healing, soothing, and sedative qualities.

Taken by itself, passionflower triggers mild euphoria when smoked or ingested, however, even in high doses it is not a strong entheogenic. Some users have reported slight visual shifts, but most commonly the main effect is a euphoric sedation.

Ajo Sacha *(mansoa alliacea)*

Ajo sacha, also known as 'forest garlic' has the scent of garlic due to its high sulphur content. At some retreats, it is given as a tea before ceremony. It is very protective and supportive, and it is sometimes added into the Ayahuasca brew itself.

It is used to calm and ground the mind, which is very useful when working with Ayahuasca as it can leave you feeling a bit ungrounded and anxious. It also works as an anti-inflammatory, cleans the blood, and uplifts your mood.

As a plant teacher, ajo sacha fortifies the immune system and gives your body more strength. It helps you gain confidence, enabling you to face adversity with more grace. It refines your senses and has been used for this purpose by hunters for centuries. It is known to clear away negative energy and is sometimes added to enhance floral baths. It is also good for *saladera* (a pattern of bad luck).

Ajo sacha is known to give you wisdom teachings vividly through dreams. Even those who have had a hard time remembering their dreams in the past will begin to have memorable dreams using this medicine.

Ajo sacha is also a great plant to use at home before you embark on your Ayahuasca journey. It works to clarify your intentions and keep you focused on your goals. It will help remove blocks caused by insecurities and fears. It is excellent to use after your Ayahuasca experiences to help integrate and accelerate your healing processes, providing you with more powerful insights.

Holy Basil *(tulsi or albacha)*

Holy basil is a great supportive plant to use when you are working with Ayahuasca. It restores balance and harmony in the mind and body and helps strengthen against stress. It is also a great herb to use daily (weeks prior to your ceremony) to help with detoxification. In the upper regions of the Amazon, Peruvian shamanic traditions have worked with holy basil, or albacha (a slightly different strain than the one used in India called *tulsi*). they are equally potent. Holy basil is considered a master plant in Peru, where it is used in the traditional shamanic Dieta process.

Holy basil provides spiritual protection (especially as a medicinal bath). It balances the energetic body and opens spiritual channels so one may understand and receive spiritual information easily. It also purifies the mind, body, and spirit; supports mental clarity, and helps the body adapt to stress. It is also a natural anti-inflammatory and antiseptic, and is helpful for migraines, nervousness, and adrenal fatigue.

In India, holy basil (*tulsi)* is known as the queen of herbs and is worshipped. It is considered to be one of the most sacred plants in the area and it has been used in spiritual and medicinal practices for thousands of years. Because of its helpfulness, the people believe it to be the embodiment of Lakishmi, the Hindu goddess of abundance and love.

Holy basil is a very playful and powerful plant, which helps with dreams and visions. It is especially beneficial for people who do artistic work and those who practice yoga or meditation, as it opens a universe of clarity and insight. It is a very effective plant for supporting your quest for harmony and awakening.

Tree Bark Tea *(cortezas de palos)*

Using tree bark tea along with Ayahuasca is especially synergistic, deepening your healing experience. This combination clears pathways in the energetic and physical body to accelerate the cleansing process. It is more cleansing than taking Ayahuasca alone.

Motherwort *(leonurus sibiricus)*

Motherwort is a 'motherly' supportive herb which is helpful before and after Ayahuasca ceremonies. Ancient herbalists have used this herb as a tool to remove evil spirits. It helps heart conditions, including heart failure, fast or irregular heartbeat, and other heart symptoms related to anxiety. This herb also induces sedative effects, helps decrease muscle spasms, and temporarily lowers blood pressure.

Motherwort has also been shown to reduce fevers, as well as treating rheumatism and lung problems, including asthma and bronchitis. For women, it helps with menopause and postpartum depression, increases fertility, and reduces anxiety or illnesses associated with nervousness or delirium.

Motherwort is not recommended for use during your Ayahuasca ceremonial retreat experience due to the increased blood flow in the body.

Peppermint *(mentha × piperita or M. balsamea willd)*

Peppermint is one of the most soothing and calming plants in the plant kingdom making it beneficial during any Ayahuasca retreat. It is especially invigorating and refreshing when used the morning following your ceremony. It will heal and calm your nerves and improve your digestion, while eliminating stomach aches (especially if taken after a meal). It also helps with morning sickness or motion sickness.

Peppermint contains anti-inflammatory astringent compounds, which brings relief to muscle pain or cramps and reduces or eliminates headaches. It naturally reduces fevers. It works well in a bath or when taken internally as a tea. Peppermint also increases the effectiveness of other herbs or supplements.

Activated Charcoal

Activated charcoal should be in every traveler's first aid kit. It is an ancient remedy that has been used successfully for centuries in treating food poisoning, diarrhea, or upset stomach. If you are traveling to Peru from far away, diarrhea can be a problem and is a normal result from changes in the climate or in your diet as well as from the effects of purging and detoxing on Ayahuasca.

Known as a binder, activated charcoal works quickly and safely by absorbing toxins in your digestive track, binding to them, and cleansing them from your system, leaving you feeling better within an hour or two. Do not be alarmed if you see black tar-like stools coming out of you, it creates black stools, which is a normal result of its use.

Psyllium

Psyllium is another important component to carry in your first aid kit (it is easier to take in pill form as it thickens in water quickly). It works miracles for travelers who become constipated or want to cleanse away toxins from the digestive tract. Be sure to drink a lot of water when taking these (see instructions on the bottle). Psyllium is a very safe and natural way to get extra fiber in your digestive track and flush out any impurities, helping you detox more effectively before or during your sacred *Dieta* phase.

Rapé (pronounced ha-peh)

Rapé is a snuff powder made from *mapacho* tobacco (*nicotiana rustica)* and alkaline ash of other plants, including cinnamon, tonka bean, clover, banana peel, or mint. Most shaman keep the exact ingredients of their particular *rapé* a secret.

It is most often made from the sacred *mapacho,* a much stronger and cleaner version than the tobacco used in other countries (*N. tabacum*).

To the Indigenous cultures of Brazil and Peru, this sacred snuff mixture has been an important part of medicinal rituals for centuries, including prior to, or during, Ayahuasca ceremonies.

The snuff powder can be self-administered or by having one person blow the snuff into the nose of the second person through a bone or bamboo handmade pipe. It is a deeply cleansing process, which may bring on vomiting, sweating, or diarrhea, depending on the level of cleansing you need done. By purging these deep toxins, afterwards you feel much calmer and more aligned with your true self.

The benefits of *rapé* are a focused and sharpened mind, increased sense of smell (you will obtain the nose of a jaguar), decalcification, and cleansing of the pineal gland, a cleansing of the energetic field from bad or negative energies, and detoxification of any parasites that may be in your body. It clears the sinuses of mucus and bacteria, which helps prevent colds. It helps ground your emotions and calms the mind. It can be effective when used with other treatments for mental illness and addictions.

Chapter 7

What to Pack

"The clearest way into the universe is through a forest wilderness"

— *John Muir*

What to Pack for the Amazon Jungle

- **Sunscreen:** Chose one with as many natural ingredients as possible.
- **Sunglasses**
- **Ear plugs:** The jungle is loud at night and you may have to share your space with someone who snores. They are also useful for sleeping on the plane.
- **Eye mask:** Useful for better sleep in the jungle and on the plane
- **Sanitary antiseptic wipes:** These are great to have on hand to help stay clean and fresh during your travels and to protect yourself from germs.
- **Bug spray:** Lemon or eucalyptus oil are good natural choices.
- **Bio-degradable soap, toothpaste, lotion, and shampoo**
- **Medicines:** Only those compatible with the medicine or to take after you leave.
- **Vitamins and supplements:** Do not bring any supplements or vitamins as they often have additives, which can interfere with Ayahuasca. To be safe, only bring what is listed in the *Supportive Plants* Chapter.
- **First aid kit:** Include a small rain poncho

- **One or two books:** Keep it light
- **Notebook and pen:** For journaling, drawing, and taking notes during workshops
- **A musical instrument**
- **A small zipped sachet:** Filled with sage, *palo santo*, Florida water, and some *mapacho* cigarettes (you can get these in Peru), a headlamp, and a lighter. It is best to have all in one sachet so you can find these things easily during ceremony.
- **Small canteen:** For hot tea for after your ceremony.
- **For women:** The Venus cup is highly recommended for your stay in Peru or other countries where they have limited septic systems. Even the washable pads can be a problem as your laundry may only be done once a week and you may not be able to dry them well enough.

Clothing for the Amazon Jungle

Bring light colored clothing as bugs are attracted to darker colors. You can also find *permethrin* treated clothing which also helps repel bugs.

- **Wide brimmed hat**: One which will keep the sun off your face and neck.
- **Bandanna and hair bands**
- **T-shirts**
- **Loose-fitting water-resistant pants for hiking**
- **Shorts:** Water-resistant hiking pants with zip-off legs that turn into shorts are the best.
- **Sturdy Teva style sandals:** For shower, sauna, rivers, lakes, or hot tubs.

- **Light bathrobe or beach shirt**: For swimming, retreat showers or spa facilities.
- **Sarong or wrap**
- **Sturdy water-resistant hiking shoes**
- **Rain poncho or rain jacket:** A light very well-ventilated breathable jacket.
- **Rain boots:** Find ones that are loose around your calves and breathable for the warm jungle environment. It is important to bring some material to cover the gap on the top part of the boot to prevent leeches or other bugs from getting inside.
- **Umbrella**
- **Day bags:** These work great to separate your clothes and keep them dry. It works even better if you can put silica canisters inside of them.
- **Smaller back pack for day hikes:** With a waterproof detachable shell.
- **Mosquito netting:** You can even buy a full-on mosquito net suit (which covers your whole body and head) for extra protection against biting flies and mosquitos (malaria prevention). Biting flies can be an even more annoying problem than the mosquitos. Mosquito netting can also be very useful to cover your bed if the retreat does not provide one.

Electronics in the Amazon jungle

The jungle is obviously full of humidity and moisture. Once you are there, you will quickly see how vital it will be to keep your clothing and electronics as dry as possible using the methods below.

- **Moisture absorbing silica gel packets or canisters:** Make sure to put enough of these in your dry packs and zip lock bags to help absorb moisture to protect your electronics and clothes. Also keep in mind they can only absorb so much moisture and will eventually stop working. So be sure to keep extra on hand in separate zip lock bags. For extra protection, you can buy ordinary silica cat litter and fill up an old sock or fabric bag.

- **Dry bags:** Keep your electronics inside zip lock baggies inside your dry bags for extra protection and to keep moisture out. It is also a great way to organize and separate everything in your suitcase.

- **Zip lock bags:** Separate everything inside your dry bags with zip lock bags and then add silica packs. This will make your life in the jungle a much happier place!

- **Camera**: Use rechargeable batteries if possible. Bring extra AA batteries for back up if your camera accepts those. (Remember to take the batteries back home with you).

- **Rechargeable batteries and charger**

- **Portable charger:** Including USB and/or other adaptors.

- **Plug adapter:** Peru uses different plugs for electronics.

- **Plastic shell form-fitting camera rain and dust cover:** Protect your camera when shooting in the wet jungle.

- **MP3 player:** For listening to meditations, books, music, or talks.

- **Laptop or notebook:** If you need to transfer documents for high-speed access in the city, bring a flash drive with you so you can transfer documents to the local computers in the city.

- **Flash drive:** Save everything in case your laptop stops working or gets stolen.

- **Alarm clock:** A small rechargeable battery operated one, or a watch.

- **Flashlight:** Hand-crank, or solar types are best.
- **Clip-on light or headlamp with a red-light option or red tape to cover the light:** The red light is important so you do not blind people in ceremonies as your eyes will become extra sensitive to light.
- **Battery operated fan:** A fan is golden in the jungle heat, especially when you are trying to sleep at night. OPOLAR portable fan is the most powerful one I have found, which comes with a handy USB rechargeable adapter.

What to Pack for The Sacred Valley

- **Sunscreen:** Chose one with as many natural ingredients as possible.
- **Sunglasses**
- **Ear plugs:** The jungle is loud at night and you may have to share your space with someone who snores. They are also useful for sleeping on the plane.
- **Eye mask:** Useful for better sleep in the jungle and on the plane
- **Sanitary antiseptic wipes:** These are great to have on hand to help stay clean and fresh during your travels and to protect yourself from germs.
- **Bug spray:** Lemon or eucalyptus oil are good natural choices.
- **Bio-degradable soap, toothpaste, lotion, and shampoo**
- **Medicines:** Only those compatible with the medicine or to take after you leave.
- **Vitamins and supplements:** Do not bring any supplements or vitamins as they often have additives, which can interfere with Ayahuasca. To be safe, only bring what is listed in the *Supportive Plants* Chapter.

- **First aid kit:** Include a small rain poncho
- **One or two books:** Keep it light
- **Notebook and pen:** For journaling, drawing, and taking notes during workshops
- **A musical instrument**
- **A small zipped sachet:** Filled with sage, palo santo, Florida water, and some *mapacho* cigarettes (you can get these in Peru), a headlamp, and a lighter. It is best to have all in one sachet so you can find these things easily during ceremony.
- **Small canteen:** For hot tea for after your ceremony.
- **For women:** The Venus cup is highly recommended for your stay in Peru or other countries where they have limited septic systems. Even the washable pads can be a problem as your laundry may only be done once a week and you may not be able to dry them well enough.

Clothing for the Sacred Valley

Prepare to dress for all climates; it can get very hot during the day, and then cold at night in this region. Also, there can be lots of gnats along the rivers or lakes. Bring light colored clothing, as bugs are attracted to darker colors.

- **Sweatshirt or sweater and warm jacket:** Keep it minimal, yet warm enough for those cold nights.
- **Umbrella and raincoat:** Light, water-resistant breathable jacket that will keep you warm on a cool evening or during a sudden downpour yet can be stuffed away or worn loosely on a warm day.
- **Wide brimmed hat**: One which will keep the sun off your face and neck.
- **Bandanna, hair bands**

- **T-shirts**
- **Loose-fitting water-resistant pants for hiking**
- **Shorts:** Water-resistant hiking pants with zip-off legs that turn into shorts are the best.
- **Sturdy Teva style sandals:** For shower, sauna, rivers, lakes, or hot tubs.
- **Light bathrobe or beach shirt**: For swimming, retreat showers or spa facilities.
- **Sarong or wrap**
- **Sturdy water-resistant hiking shoes**
- **Rain poncho or rain jacket:** A light very well-ventilated breathable jacket.
- **Rain boots:** Find ones that are loose around your calves and breathable for the warm jungle environment. It is important to bring some material to cover the gap on the top part of the boot to prevent leeches or other bugs from getting inside.
- **Umbrella**
- **Day bags:** These work great to separate your clothes and keep them dry. It works even better if you can put silica canisters inside of them.
- **Smaller back pack for day hikes:** With a waterproof detachable shell.
- **Mosquito netting:** You can even buy a full-on mosquito net suit (which covers your whole body and head) for extra protection against biting flies and mosquitos (malaria prevention). Biting flies can be an even more annoying problem than the mosquitos. Mosquito netting can also be very useful to cover your bed if the retreat does not provide one.

Electronics in the Sacred Valley

The Sacred Valley during the rainy season is the only time you really have to be concerned with taking extra steps to protect your electronics from moisture.

- **Moisture absorbing silica gel packets or canisters:** Make sure to put enough of these in your dry packs and zip lock bags to help absorb moisture to protect your electronics and clothes. Also keep in mind they can only absorb so much moisture and will eventually stop working. So be sure to keep extra on hand in separate zip lock bags. For extra protection, you can buy ordinary silica cat litter and fill up an old sock or fabric bag.

- **Dry bags:** Keep your electronics inside zip lock baggies inside your dry bags for extra protection and to keep moisture out. It is also a great way to organize and separate everything in your suitcase.

- **Zip lock bags:** Separate everything inside your dry bags with zip lock bags and then add silica packs. This will make your life in the jungle a much happier place!

- **Camera**: Use rechargeable batteries if possible. Bring extra AA batteries for back up if your camera accepts those. (Remember to take the batteries back home with you).

- **Rechargeable batteries and charger**

- **Portable charger:** Including USB and/or other adaptors.

- **Plug adapter:** Peru uses different plugs for electronics.

- **Plastic shell form-fitting camera rain and dust cover:** Protect your camera when shooting in the wet jungle.

- **MP3 player:** For listening to meditations, books, music, or talks.

- **Laptop or notebook:** If you need to transfer documents for high-speed access in the city, bring a flash drive with you so you can transfer documents to the local computers in the city.

- **Flash drive:** Save everything in case your laptop stops working or gets stolen.

- **Alarm clock:** A small rechargeable battery operated one, or a watch.

- **Flashlight:** Hand-crank, or solar types are best.

- **Clip-on light or headlamp with a red-light option or red tape to cover the light:** The red light is important so you do not blind people in ceremonies as your eyes will become extra sensitive to light.

- **Battery operated fan:** A fan is golden in the jungle heat, especially when you are trying to sleep at night. OPOLAR portable fan is the most powerful one I have found, which comes with a handy USB rechargeable adapter.

- **Blood oxygen meter:** For altitude and to check your heart rate.

Money

- **Spending money:** For day trips, excursions, and shopping for souvenirs. South America is a cash driven society.

- **$500 minimum extra money for medical emergencies:** Most places out of the country will not accept money from your home country, so be sure to convert your money to *soles*.

- **Cash:** In Peru, they are very particular to the condition of your money. They will only accept clean crisp bills. Anything wrinkled or even with a small tear in it will most likely be rejected. Bring small bills. Large bills above $10 are hard to exchange, so do not bring $50s or $100s with you unless you are staying for a long time. (You are limited to $10,000 at the airport). They are very cautious about counterfeit bills, so it is very difficult to exchange large bills into smaller amounts unless you have a local bank account. If you must bring large bills or a lot of money, no larger than $20s is best.

ATM, Credit Cards, Travelers Checks, and Cash

- **ATM card:** Your card may not work in another country. Make sure you have enough cash in case you have problems. Also, be sure to call your bank ahead of time and let them know where you are travelling to avoid problems, as they may think your card was stolen and freeze your account.

- **Traveler's checks:** usually has a 20-day hold, if you can even find a place to cash them. You normally need to deposit them in an account for them to clear and so you would need to open a bank account.

- **Credit cards:** will not work in many places and usually include high overseas fees if they do work. They normally only work at expensive tourist hotels and resorts. Call your credit card bank ahead of time and let them know where you are travelling to avoid problems as it is a giant red flag for them when your credit card is used in another country. Avoid having your account getting frozen.

Cell Phones

Your cell phone is unlikely to work in most areas of South America unless you have a satellite phone. You might want to check with your carrier to find out if your cell phone will work where you are going. Sometimes they do; sometimes they do not. It depends on whether the technology of the phone matches the same technology as the cell towers in your destination country. However, it may cost as much as $3 a minute with your cell phone carrier in your home country, so you may be better off using local cheaper methods of calling home.

Another option is to purchase a cheap local cell phone, which features a phone number chip (SIM) or, if you already have an unlocked phone, you can insert a locally purchased SIM card. You can purchase phone cards *(saldo)* and make your calls as needed. You can even call overseas on these phones inexpensively and your loved ones will be able to call you too. Phone calls to other countries are not expensive in most places in South America.

What NOT to Bring

Disposable batteries: Unless you want to carry them back with you, so you can dispose of them properly. Disposing of batteries properly in South America is very difficult. Bring solar powered, hand-cranked, or rechargeable battery flashlights with you. Adapters are normally not needed in South America if you are using USA electronics.

Airline Tips

Call each airline on which you are traveling to check the baggage weight and size limits. You do not want to have to throw out precious luggage or pay high fees for extra weight unnecessarily.

Visa Requirements

In 2019 Peru changed the requirements for visitors. You must now ask for a six-month visa. You are not permitted to exceed this maximum stay in a single trip.

Avoid Altitude Sickness Naturally

- Iquitos: 341 feet
- Pucallpa: 505 feet
- Lima: 5,080 feet
- Machu Picchu: 8,040 feet

- Ollantaytambo: 9,150 feet
- Urubamba: 9,420 feet
- Calca: 9,606 feet
- Pisac: 9,751 feet
- Cusco: 11,152 feet

Altitude sickness generally starts affecting people at 8,000 feet. If you are going to a higher elevation, you can acclimate better by staying in a lower altitude area for a while. For example, if you are going to the Sacred Valley, it is not a good idea to stay in Cusco right away as the altitude there is much higher than surrounding areas.

Other ways to help with altitude sickness are to avoid alcohol and drink lots of extra water. Take it easy by not walking around or exercising too much the first day or two.

Chlorophyll drops or chlorophyll soft gel capsules are a natural alternative solution to the normally prescribed *Diamox.* Chlorophyll is highly effective; buy some before you leave home to have on hand. Take some soft gel capsules or put a few drops in your water daily. Chlorophyll increases the amount of red blood cells in your system. The more red-blood cells there are, the more oxygen can be absorbed, which greatly reduces the effects of altitude sickness.

You may want to consider getting a **blood oxygen meter.** Your blood oxygen level (SP02) should not fall below ninety percent. By bringing one of these along, you can easily check where you are, and if it falls below the ideal level, you can lie down and take a break. Take in some deep breaths, listen to your body, and make sure it is okay before you move on. This meter can also check your heart rate, which is good for those who have heart problems.

About the Author

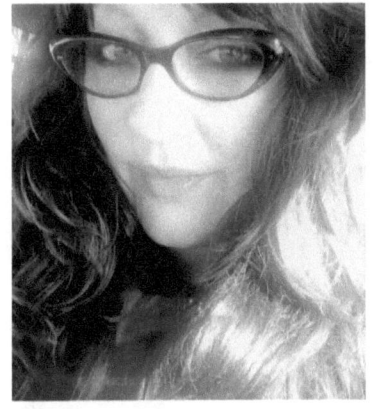

Sharon C. Davis grew up in Milwaukee, Wisconsin. In 1996, she moved to Boulder, Colorado, where she studied at the *Boulder College of Massage*, becoming a Certified Massage Therapist (CMT). In 2005, she received a Bachelor of Arts in Multimedia and Web Design from *The Art Institute of Denver, Colorado.*

In 2010 she began to have mysterious health issues which conventional medical doctors were unable to diagnose. Thus, began her journey into alternative methods of healing. She finally discovered, seven years later, that she was suffering from chronic Lyme disease.

After extensive research, including consultation with Naturopaths, herbalists, and shaman, she found herself on a journey with Ayahuasca and other healing plant medicines. Sharon became an expert in herbs, sacred plant medicines, and alternative healing in her efforts to heal herself holistically.

Sharon practices Kundalini yoga, Vajrayana Buddhism and meditation, which she finds to be a crucial base for providing spiritual awareness, consciousness, and strength for Ayahuasca and other Sacred Medicine journeys.

Additionally, she is working toward traveling throughout South America, offering her advertising and marketing services to spiritual healing retreats to raise awareness in order to help others heal both physically and spiritually with Ayahuasca.

With this book, she hopes to help others by delivering an accurate picture of preparation for Ayahuasca so that they may be able to experience the best circumstances for personal healing and raise awareness of our need to heal the planet as well.

Sharon C. Davis
Web & Print Designer
Photographer
Holistic Practitioner

www.exposedpixel.com
www.sacredsagehealing.com

Notes

The Ayahuasca Guidebook

www.ingramcontent.com/pod-product-compliance
Lightning Source LLC
Chambersburg PA
CBHW031249280526
45784CB00004B/1774